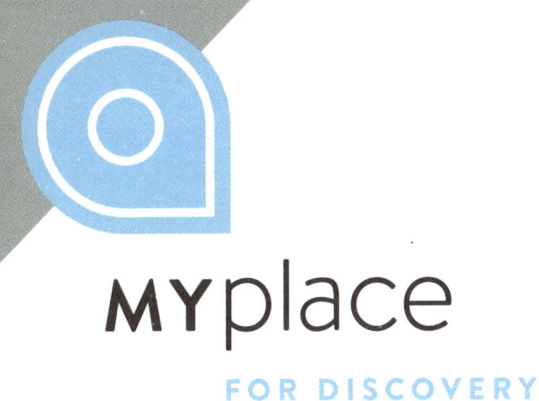

MYplace

FOR DISCOVERY

Published by First Place for Health
Galveston, Texas, USA
www.firstplaceforhealth.com
Printed in the USA
© 2018 First Place for Health

Cover design by Faceout Studio, Tim Green
Interior print design by Faceout Studio, Amanda Kreutzer

ISBN 978-1-942425-26-7

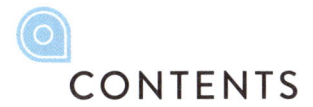

CONTENTS

MY PLACE FOR DISCOVERY: BOOK ONE

Searching Myself

MY PLACE FOR DISCOVERY

This book is the first of a four-part series from the First Place for Health wellness program. As you work through these questions and exercises, you will begin to understand your eating and health habits more clearly. Our goal is to be unafraid as we explore our deepest self. We want to discover why we make the health decisions we make and to uncover the unconscious behaviors that have led to our health issues, including weight, strength, flexibility, disease, and much more.

Human beings have struggled with behavior since the beginning of time. In the Garden, Adam and Eve made a disobedient choice to eat the wrong food. Throughout history others chose the wrong path, too. Even while fiercely following God, Moses, Noah, Samson, and others disobeyed and failed. Finally, King David cried out, "Search me, O God, and know my heart . . ."

In modern history, groups such as AA, Celebrate Recovery, and others have developed twelve steps to help a person delve into the reasons why he or she chooses alcohol or drugs or food to satisfy deep psychological voids.

The FP4H *My Place for Discovery* program will help you take that kind of fearless moral inventory from a spiritual point of view. While some of the issues we face are psychological, medical, or personal issues, FP4H does not claim to be doctors, psychologists, or counselors, and we are not equipped to give clinical care to those with deep psychological or medical issues.

However, FP4H—and you—have the most powerful tool of all to deal with these and other issues: the Word of God.

The majority of us don't need medical or clinical help—because we have a physical problem with a spiritual answer.

The spiritual expertise we need is found in the Word. So *My Place for Discovery* is written to help you identify what may lead you to overeat, and we'll point you in the direction of an answer from God.

Your personal *My Place for Discovery* project centers around four books to be used in conjunction with four different 12-week FP4H sessions. Each book will take twelve weeks to complete and follows the pattern of your FP4H Bible study; but instead of working through a daily lesson as you do in your Bible study, you will only complete one lesson per week in *My Place for Discovery*.

We've kept the *My Place for Discovery* weekly lesson at a practical length so that you will have plenty of time to go deep into your memory, heart, and feelings. One lesson per week will allow plenty of time to work through these personal subjects.

We are excited about the changes that *My Place for Discovery* will make for you.

A WORD FROM THE AUTHOR

When I started writing the *My Place for Discovery* project, I was excited about building a tool for FP4H, but I didn't know that God would make a spectacular change in me.

I have always loved sugary food—cookies, cakes, pudding, and especially ice cream. And if the delicacy was chocolate, I loved it even more. My affection wasn't slight or simple like someone who merely enjoyed a sweet occasionally. No, my affection was a serious addiction. Ice cream called my name from the freezer. I felt compelled to eat cookies until the package was empty. I learned to bake the most luscious desserts. I loved sugar.

I would be ashamed for you to know how many sweets I could eat or how much I ate when I knew no one was looking. I had a theory: If no one saw me eat it, the calories didn't count. On top of my physical desire and love for sugar, I used it to ease my emotional pain, because for me, sugar satisfied me when life hurt. In his book *Sugar Nation*, Jeff O'Connell said, "Sugar gave rise to the slave trade; now sugar has enslaved us." I am an example of being a slave to the sweet stuff.

Then, as I researched the topics in this book, I took a new look at my assets and flaws and considered underlying feelings of selfishness, anger, and negativity that I didn't know were hidden in my heart. I caught a glimpse of my addiction to sugar and a vision of the power of God to overcome my bad choices, habits, and obsessions.

God changed me dramatically.

I do not crave sweets now. Imagine the miracle! I'm free to eat sweets and I take a bite sometimes, but the bite is all I want. I push the dessert plate away after a meal. No creamy sweet treat is calling my name. My friends are surprised, and my family is astonished. There is no way to describe the change in me except to declare that God has done a miracle.

I can't wait to go through the book again and again so that God can continue to change my heart, mind, and behavior. You can win the battle over disobedience, poor food choices, and habits, too.

Let's begin by praying, "O Lord, search me."

Karen Porter

ABOUT THE AUTHOR

Karen Porter is a national and international speaker and the author of six books including *Speak Like Jesus* and *I'll Bring the Chocolate* and her latest, *If you Give a Girl a Giant*.

Karen is the founder of *kae* Creative Solutions, a communications consulting firm and the co-owner of Bold Vision Books, a traditional publishing company. She coaches aspiring writers and speakers and teaches on the national staff of CLAS-Seminars. She serves on the Board of Directors for several non-profit organizations such as CLASSeminars, First Place for Health, and Advanced Writers and Speakers Association.

Karen considers her marriage to George as her greatest achievement. In her spare time, she continues her life-long quest to find the perfect purse.

CHAPTER ONE: UNDERSTANDING THE *MY PLACE FOR DISCOVERY* PROJECT

In more than 30 years of ministry, we at FP4H have watched thousands of men and women find balance in the four areas of life that Jesus mentioned in Luke 10:27—spiritual, emotional, mental, and physical. Those in the program have learned to manage the spiritual side of life by spending daily time with God and through the Bible studies of FP4H. We have identified our emotional eating triggers and have tried to cope with them. We have exercised our brains by learning memory verses. We have followed the Live It food plan and have discovered that food is good and is provided in abundance by our God. We have learned that some foods aren't the best for us individually, even though others may be able to enjoy that food without consequence. We've also learned that not eating some foods or eating certain foods in moderation is our best healthy choice.

And thousands have lost weight; many have kept it off.

Approaching our health and wellness goals in this four-sided-person manner has helped us find equilibrium in the middle of busyness. We have learned to eat healthy, exercise wisely, seek God constantly, set our mind on powerful goals, and put aside mindless emotional habits. For many, the discoveries made and implemented in FP4H have been life saving and live giving. Others however, haven't found the freedom to live within the bounty of God or the ability to live in balance. In fact, more than two-thirds of us continue in the program, going to class, completing the Bible study questions, following some of the guidelines for eating, and sometimes beating the emotional forces that plague us. But we haven't succeeded at losing and keeping off the weight, and we aren't living in freedom. Even those who have lost large amounts of weight aren't always free—rigidly and obsessively trying to keep up with the food plan and exercise program.

So we've asked ourselves, "Why?"

We know the program is valid and well rounded. We know the Bible studies are solid and practical and helpful. We have the tools and the methods. Why aren't we all at our goal weight? Is there some inherent structural flaw in how we tackle our goals? Why aren't we free?

Freedom

Freedom is a powerful word. FP4H board member Gari Meacham says, "We have a living hope for freedom, not merely behavior modification or another food and exercise plan."

Jesus said, "So if the son sets you free, you will be free indeed"

—John 8:36

The dictionary presents some interesting facts about freedom: that it is exemption from external control or regulation; that independence is the power to determine action without restraint; that autonomy is the opposite of bondage or slavery. Are those descriptions a picture of your wellness? Are you exempt from regulation—eating what you want to eat when you are hungry? Are you able to enjoy food without placing severe boundaries or restraints on yourself? Are you a slave to food—either what to eat or what not to eat? It is possible to be in bondage to good food (obsessed with measuring and ingredients and percentages) as well as bad food (overeating sugar or full-fat dairy or junk food).

True freedom in wellness is eating what you like in healthy proportions and moving your body because you love the activity and the strength. Bondage, on the other hand, is out-of-control eating and sedentary living. The opposite behavior—eating nothing you like and over-exercising because of fear—also breeds bondage.

So be free.

We like those words. We'd love to be free. And thin.

Unfortunately, the word "free" also has a negative effect for some of us. If I say, "I'm free," my heart sings with the idea. But my song is not of liberty; it is of license. You too? We like the idea of unrestricted, spontaneous, uncontrolled permissive living.

But that's what got us here in the first place.

So how do we get to that center place of liberty, that hub of the wheel that is named freedom? There has to be some reason I am stuck. Why do I continually go to my FP4H classes and try hard to lose weight and yet never live in freedom? Never develop an intimate personal relationship with Him? Never conquer my fears and/or change my mindset? I know God is offering freedom, yet I take the license as permission to go my unhealthy way.

My Place for Discovery

We have added the *My Place for Discovery* component to FP4H because we all want victory. These small books will help us go deeper—physically, spiritually, mentally, emotionally—and live free.

Think about it. We have come to FP4H because we want to live in wellness. We have discovered the four-sided person. The Bible studies are powerful and life-changing. The Live It plan works. The emotional mapping, personality profiles, and lifestyle analysis have taken us deeper into why we overeat. Memorizing verses has helped our minds stay alert and centered on the Word. We've even told others about the program and its advantages. But we can't seem to go beyond these surface levels of the four-sided person. It's as if we packed for a trip but lost our luggage.

There is more. There are tools that will take us to the next level. And this *My Place for Discovery* project is designed to help us go there.

Comparison to Sanctification

Perhaps we could liken our dilemma to the pattern of a believer in the walk of faith. Consider Andrea. She attended a Bible study in her friend's home. That day's lesson helped her realize the sinful condition of her heart as she heard about the salvation offered by Jesus. She accepted His mercy and grace and became a Christ follower. She began attending church, making better life choices, resisting sin, and choosing to make moral decisions. Then she learned how to witness and dutifully began telling the world about Christ.

This pattern is typical. But Andrea soon discovered a gap between becoming a Christ follower and becoming a witness. She had not grown in her faith, nor had she developed the kind of deep intimacy with God that changes mindsets and builds wisdom and strength. Discouragement set in and she felt as if she was simply going through the motions. She had not reached that quiet, assured place where a person knows the mind of God—that place where you not only have God, but also He has you.

In theological terms, this "gap" is called sanctification—the growth, the changing, the transforming. It is the place where your beliefs and your actions are in sync—not to make the choice to live a holy life, but living a holy life because that is who you are.

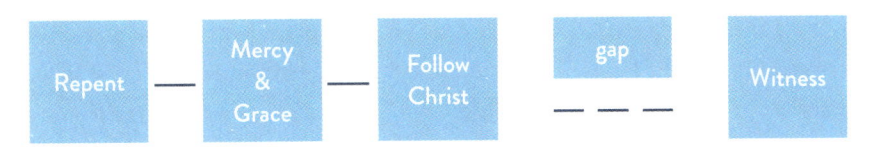

The focus of justification (our salvation and rescue from sin) is the removal of the guilt (and punishment) of sin. Sanctification is found as we make progress toward being like Him (see 1 John 3:2). We have been transformed, we will be transformed, and we are being transformed (see 2 Corinthians 3:18). The sanctified life is victorious (see Romans 8:37) even though it is lived in the context of temptation and suffering.

There is no quick fix in sanctification, no instant victory, no sudden freedom. We long for it because we belong to Christ, but we must follow Him to do it. The sanctification process requires us to undress and re-dress. We must put off the old, put on the new (see Colossians 3:5-14). Our new clothes are compassion, kindness, humility, gentleness, and patience. In these new clothes, we can forgive and love, and grow in the grace and knowledge of our Lord and Savior Jesus Christ (see Ephesians 4:22-24; 2 Peter 3:18).

And while the concept of sanctification is a theological term and is acquired through spiritual devotion and apprenticeship to Jesus, there is a similar gap in our journey to wellness and health.

The Missing Gap in Wellness

We began the FP4H journey because we realized we were not in a healthy place. Maybe we saw that all-time highest number ever on the scale, or the doctor shocked us into understanding that we needed to get healthy. Maybe we heard the word "obese" for the first time as it related to us personally. Maybe we went to the closet and had nothing to wear, because everything was too small. Maybe we tried to chase a child or grandchild and fell breathlessly into a chair, unable to keep up. That dark-night place brought an understanding of our need for help.

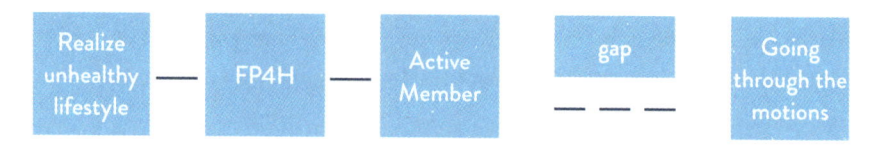

And then we heard about FP4H. This program promised to guide us to the freedom of healthy living. We joined up and in. We did the activities and Bible studies and tried to follow the food plan. We even lost some weight. We committed. But somewhere along the way, discouragement or reality set in, and we aren't really following the program anymore. We still work through the Bible studies, and we love to go to the meetings. We see the help that God offers, but we don't extend our hand to Him, and we don't succeed. We hear others' weight-loss stories, and we long for it to be our story too. Something hinders us and puts us in the gap between starting well and finishing victoriously.

What is that something? What are the hindrances?

Strongholds

A stronghold is a place of refuge or defense. I can find safety there. I can hide from my enemies. I can protect myself. It is a hideout, a fort, a guard tower. Yet that place of refuge can become a prison. I cannot get out of the stronghold, which holds power over me. Though I went there first as a place of safety, I stay there because I am powerless over the grip it has on me.

Someone told Maryanne what Joellen said. It hurt to realize that her best friend wasn't loyal and would say such a hurtful thing. So Maryanne retreated into the safety of her family and home. She baked bread and cookies to create a feeling of warmth and love. She didn't answer phone calls or emails and her withdrawal became a prison. Her separation destroyed the joy of friendship. So, for consolation, she baked more and ate more.

Marla wanted to be a success in her career, so she worked harder than anyone else in the office, laboring long hours, and devoting all her energy to the job. She reached the success she craved and it felt like a powerful place until she realized she had sacrificed relationships with family and friends to get to the top. So now she buys expensive gifts and toys for her family and takes them to fancy restaurants to try to repair the relationships. Her life and health are out of balance.

When your self-esteem is at an all-time low because of the weight you've gained and then you overhear someone mention your weight gain, the hurt of that remark causes you to say you don't care. So you isolate yourself from those people. The isolation makes you feel even worse about yourself, so you eat your favorite snacks and desserts to compensate. And the cycle of hate-myself eating begins and seems to never end.

In 2 Corinthians 10:4, the word translated "strongholds" in English comes from a word in the Greek language that is a metaphor for "arguments and every proud obstacle to the knowledge of God."

What do I argue about? What makes me so proud, so sure I'm right? For some of us, it is our knowledge of the Bible or how much doctrine we know. For some, it is a bent of personality—we are strong and sure. For others, our pride stronghold is how well we raised our kids or how beautiful our home is. Pride comes in all flavors—from pride in losing weight to pride that I don't care about weight. It comes from living independently without restraints or from rigidly orchestrating every moment.

But no matter where I'm holed up in my stronghold, Jesus must become my new refuge. He is where I must run when I'm feeling trapped or when failure overwhelms me.

Remember, our battle is spiritual.

For though we walk in the flesh, we are not waging war according to the flesh. For the weapons of our warfare are not of the flesh but have divine power to destroy strongholds. We destroy arguments and every lofty opinion raised against the knowledge of God, and take every thought captive to obey Christ, being ready to punish every disobedience, when your obedience is complete

—2 Corinthians 10:3-6

Our battles are not earthly; we can't use earthly weapons, strategies, or tactics.

- **Earthly weapons**—fad-diet plans, lose-weight-quick schemes, cardboard food, pills, shakes, etc.

- **Mental strategies**—mind over matter, "I'll force myself," hypnosis, positive thinking, self-talk.

- **Emotional tactics**—crying, whining, or a cavalier attitude of "I don't care about my looks. I just wanna have fun!"

Our battle is spiritual. We need spiritual weapons and plans and strategies and skills.

Our armor is the armor that God provides (see Ephesians 6:14-17); and with that armor, He gives us practical solutions to our weight problem, solutions that are based in truth. Food is good, and we can enjoy it. A balanced plan for the four-sided person allows us to meet our emotional, physical, mental, and spiritual needs. This balance includes eating good food in reasonable quantities, moving our body to preserve muscle tone and strength, searching for the traps that cause us to fail in eating and exercising, and discovering God's role in all these areas of day-to-day life.

The battle is why FP4H has developed the *My Place for Discovery* project. Although physiologists and psychologists have reviewed and approved the FP4H program, we do not seek to offer solutions from the medical or psychological realms. We believe our emotions and feelings don't reflect our external reality, instead they reflect our internal reality.[1] We believe we have a physical problem with a spiritual solution. Some issues cannot be perceived by the five senses because they are only seen through the Holy Spirit's eyes.[2] At FP4H our expertise is spiritual, because we have the Word of God, which gives us answers to our dilemma.

All Scripture is breathed out by God and profitable for teaching, for reproof, for correction, and for training in righteousness, that the man of God may be complete, equipped for every good work

—2 Timothy 3:16

Our power comes from God.

So let's begin searching for those difficulties that keep us from accessing His power in our health pursuits.

This book contains one lesson for each week of your FP4H session. It is a supplement and a companion to your Bible study. Work through one each week and be ready to discuss the lesson in your FP4H class meeting.

CHAPTER TWO: ACKNOWLEDGING DISOBEDIENCE

The Bible explains that God knew everything about Jeremiah. He knew the man's parents and his heritage, and God called Jeremiah to preach as a prophet to the nations. God even set Jeremiah apart and appointed him before Jeremiah was born. Jeremiah's life was planned and anointed, but God asked the man to obey. Obedience matters to God.

Jeremiah whined, "I'm too young and inexperienced." God answered, "Don't say that! Go where I send you. Say what I tell you to say. And do not be afraid."

Every man and woman comes to the place of decision when God asks us to be obedient, just as He asked Jeremiah. Will we say yes to what He has planned for us? Write a prayer asking God to help you become obedient.

_____

_____

_____

_____

Jesus said, "If you love me, you will obey me because you love me." Jesus never asks us to do anything that would harm us. He doesn't make mistakes. If we believe, He is pleased. But if we hesitate or refuse to obey, it shows our unbelief. What I do reveals what I believe about God. My best reaction is always obedience because obedience pleases God.

Temptation

Food was the original instrument of temptation that the enemy used with mankind. When the serpent approached Eve, he pointed out the luscious fruit on the forbidden tree. The fruit wasn't necessary for Eve's diet or nutrition, because the garden was full of food. When she saw how good the fruit looked, she desired it, and then she took it—and in that action she disobeyed God.

Our disobedience is the enemy's success. It's no wonder he still uses food to tempt us.

That day Eve tried to hide her disobedience. Have you tried to hide your disobedience concerning food in any of these ways?

- o I go through the drive-thru window when I'm alone.

- o I say I'm not hungry when with a group, then eat at home to make up for it.

- o I wear a size larger than I need so that my clothes will look as if I've lost weight.

- o I eat to avoid uncomfortable situations or conversations.

- o No one approves of me anyway, so I eat.

- o I hide food around the house.

We've even learned to hide behind our physical appearance as if it is a shield. Even though we may feel guilt or shame, we cope with our disobedience by saying that we don't care how we look or feel. The key to obedience is hearing God. The best way to hear from God is to spend time with Him daily, not only talking to Him in prayer, but also listening to Him by reading His Word and by hearing the Holy Spirit.

Do you have a certain time to sit with your Bible in the presence of God? If so, when? If not, when would be a good time for you?

_____

_____

_____

_____

_____

Do you have a certain place you always go to when you spend time with God? If so, where? If not, where in your home would be a good spot?

_____

_____

_____

_____

_____

_____

What is your normal routine for a quiet time? Describe what you do, such as read a Bible passage, read a devotional book, pray, journal, sing, etc.

_____

_____

_____

_____

_____

_____

_____

_____

Spending time with God is the key that opens the door to intimacy. The threshold of that door is radical obedience. We must hear Him, and we must also obey. Action is the proof of obedience.

What is God asking you to do in these areas of life?

Family _____

_____

Finances _____

_____

Eating _____

_____

Exercising _____

_____

FP4H _____

_____

Serving others _____

_____

Overeating Equals Disobedience

We know overeating isn't good for us. It harms more than our health; it also destroys our relationship with God. Most of us haven't thought of overeating as disobedience to God. Why? Because we don't think of our food habits as spiritual. But when we are focused on food, the fixation takes over every other life decision—from planning the next meal or snack to worrying about whether we ate too much or if we ate the right foods. We've tried diets and schemes, but we can't stop overeating—until we see it as a sin issue and realize it is disobedience.

We can deny that we are disobedient. We can blame someone else; but in the end, we are responsible for our choices. And if the choice is overeating, whether to derive pleasure or because we can't seem to stop eating, we are not putting God in first place and we are not listening to His will for our body. Overeating does not please God because we tend to worship food and make it an idol. We overeat because it makes us feel good. The Bible puts gluttony (overeating) and alcohol abuse in the same category (see Proverbs 23:21). It is never good to let some substance or some food gain control.

Your disobedience of overeating is harmful to your body. Check which of these ailments you have experienced:

○ High cholesterol

○ Diabetes

○ Heart disease

○ High blood pressure (hypertension)

○ Sleep apnea

○ Depression

○ Kidney disease

○   Arthritis

○   Bone deterioration

○   Knee problems

○   Hip problems

○   Stroke

These physical difficulties are often a result of untreated overeating. What does this verse say about the body?

> *Don't you realize that your body is the temple of the Holy Spirit, who lives in you and was given to you by God? You do not belong to yourself, for God bought you with a high price. So you must honor God with your body*
>
> —1 Corinthians 6:19, NLT

_____

_____

_____

_____

_____

_____

_____

Since the body is the temple or residence of the Holy Spirit, how have you prepared His home within you? What can you do to make His dwelling a better place?

_____

_____

_____

_____

_____

_____

_____

_____

_____

_____

_____

_____

_____

_____

_____

_____

Freedom includes the freedom to tell God things we cannot say aloud. Write a prayer now and confess your disobedience, asking God to give you strength and courage to obey.

_____

_____

_____

_____

_____

_____

_____

_____

_____

_____

_____

_____

_____

_____

_____

_____

_____

CHAPTER THREE: DISCOVERING MY ASSETS AND FLAWS

When an entrepreneur begins a new venture or a person needs to make a decision, it is helpful to make a list of pros and cons. Let's begin our *My Place for Discovery* project with a similar exercise by considering our personal assets and flaws. We will look at our strengths and opportunities and also study our weaknesses and threats. In business, this kind of search is called a SWOT—strengths, weaknesses, opportunities, and threats. Most people are surprised to discover that they have so many assets, but they are also likely to discover some flaws they didn't realize existed.

The reason for a search like this in FP4H is primarily to boost our confidence in the talents and abilities God gave us and to confront mistakes, limitations, vulnerabilities, and fragile areas that lead us to unhealthy habits and undermine our wellness goals. The sixteenth-century philosopher Francis Bacon said, "Knowledge is power." He was right, as was the cartoon character, GI Joe, who said, "Knowing is half the battle." If we recognize our pluses and identify our minuses, we will find solutions and remedies. The knowledge we gain from this search project will alter our responses, enabling us to think before we binge and overindulge. When stress slaps us in the face and our normal reaction would be to eat a tub of ice cream, we will be able to comprehend what is really happening in our brain and multiply our ability to counteract the urge for creamy cold sugar. We will react with flexibility instead of stubbornness. We will be realistic instead of perfectionistic. Knowledge really is power.

Assets

Circle the words that describe your assets, strengths, and opportunities. (Choose at least five.) Research shows that you likely have more than 20 wonderful assets.

Forgiving	Generous	Calm	Agreeable
Face my problems	Careful	Meticulous	Concerned

Expansive	Self-reliant	Obedient	Respectful
Real	Honest	Kind	Patient
Decisive	Flexible	Confident	Tolerant
Quiet	Realistic	Hopeful	Thrifty
Loyal	Organized	Hard-worker	Funny
Other	Other	Other	Other
_____	_____	_____	_____

As we go through this list of valuable qualities, we see many decent, respectable, worthy, and beneficial traits. In the space below, list what you consider to be your top five assets and write a sentence beside each one that describes how this strength functions in your life. For example, "Organized: My strength of organization helps me keep important papers in order and easily accessible."

1.

2.

3.

4.

5.

Now look at each strength again. How does that strength assist you in your wellness journey? For example, "Organization: My strength of organization helps me prepare healthy meals ahead of time."

1.

2.

3.

4.

5.

Strengths are assets that we can grow to benefit our life. Living within our pluses, skills, and talents allows us to manage our wellbeing. In fact, God will strengthen our strengths. "Fear not, for I am with you; be not dismayed, for I am your God; I will strengthen you, I will help you, I will uphold you with my righteous right hand" (Isaiah 41:10). Our strength is rooted in Him: "I can do all things through him who strengthens me" (Philippians 4:13, ESV).

In the space below, write a prayer asking God to help you make choices and take actions that will enhance your strengths. Be sure to mention each of the five strengths (listed above) in your prayer.

_____

_____

_____

Flaws

Now let's consider the weaknesses that cause us to give in to the addictions and indulgences that are the root of our overeating and weight gain. When we over-indulge or demand our own way, we make food an idol, but the downward spiral starts with a weak spot. Reviewing our flaws is not judging or battering or attacking. Instead, it is a realistic admission of the shortcoming and an understanding that it can be choked out of our behavior. It is recognition of the addiction, the trigger, and discovering the moment when we slip in the power of the flaw.

Circle the words that describe your flaws, weaknesses, and threats. (Choose at least five.) Remember, this exercise is not to condemn yourself or beat your-self up. Instead, it is following the example of the psalmist who cried out to God, "Search me, oh God . . ." (Psalm 139:23).

Angry	Critical	Defensive	Dependent
Agitated	Disobedient	Insolent	Exaggerator
Liar	Gossip	Greedy	Impatient
Withholding	Timid	Stubborn	Procrastinator
Argumentative	Anxious	Judgmental	Loud
Avoidant	Perfectionistic	Pessimistic	Self-contro
Careless	Victim	Wasteful	Unreliable
Sloppy	Unfeeling	Messy	Insecure
Other	Other	Other	Other

These weaknesses lead us along the wrong path, causing us to make poor choices and react inappropriately. In the space below, list what you consider to be your top five weaknesses and write a sentence beside each one that describes how this weakness functions in your life. For example, "Procrastinator: Procrastination causes me to keep important papers in piles and boxes so that I can't find them when they are needed."

1.

2.

3.

4.

5.

Now look at each weakness again. How does it hinder your wellness journey? For example, "Procrastinator: The weakness of procrastination causes me to say that I'll start following the FP4H Live It plan on Monday, but today . . ."

1.

2.

3.

4.

5.

It is possible to be dishonest about our flaws, perpetuating a fraud by exaggeration or leaving out details—so that we look better. We may love ourselves too much to look deeply enough to see any underlying imperfection. We may hate some part of ourselves or feel disappointed that we aren't all good or all perfect. We may refuse to believe we are capable of being wrong. Perhaps you evaluate every situation and every opportunity with the question "What's in it for me?" "Our fallen nature seems to believe that if enough people admire us, we just might believe we are admirable."[3] But lying to yourself or to God will not help you overcome the obstacle, and stuffing your feelings will not keep you from stuffing food.

Of the five flaws you listed, which one do you tend to be dishonest about and why?

_____

_____

_____

_____

_____

_____

_____

Honest evaluation keeps us away from cavalier attitudes such as "I don't care what anyone thinks" or "I hate myself, so why would anyone else like me?" God will help us in our weaknesses and give us strength where none existed before. Paul understood this when he wrote, "But he [God] said to me, 'My grace is sufficient for you, for my power is made perfect in weakness.' Therefore, I will boast all the more gladly of my weaknesses, so that the power of Christ may rest upon me" (2 Corinthians 12:9, ESV). In fact, God uses our weaknesses to make us stronger: "For when I am weak, then I am strong" (2 Corinthians 12:10, ESV).

In the space below, write a prayer asking God to help you make choices and take actions that will change your weaknesses to strengths or to help you turn to God in your weakness. Be sure to mention in your prayer each of the five assets and flaws that you identified.

_____

_____

_____

_____

_____

_____

_____

_____

_____

_____

_____

_____

_____

_____

_____

_____

_____

_____

_____

_____

_____

_____

_____

_____

_____

_____

_____

_____

_____

CHAPTER FOUR: EXPLORING REJECTION AND BROKEN RELATIONSHIPS

1. Name a time when you felt rejected. (You may have many rejections in your past. We suggest you explore the first one that comes to mind—no matter how trivial it may seem.)

2. Who rejected you?

3. What were the circumstances of the rejection?

4. What was said?

5. How did you respond at the time?

   - Quick back-talk such as: "You are wrong." or "You do it too." or "Don't be so mean."

   - Denial.

   - Kept quiet because you were hurt.

   - Kept quiet because you didn't want to say something you'd regret later.

6. How did you feel after the rejection?

   - Sad.

   - Angry.

   - Shattered.

   - Denied that you care.

   - Guilt—*I must have done something to deserve this.* or *What have I done to deserve this?*

7. What have you done since then to try to soothe the pain?

- ○ Removed that person from your life.

- ○ Retold the story—changing the details to make yourself look better.

- ○ Took some action that was vindictive or retaliatory.

- ○ Kept trying to reconcile and have this person back in your life.

- ○ Asked God to help you forgive and move on.

- ○ Other _____

Describe how you feel about that past rejection today.

_____

_____

_____

_____

_____

_____

_____

_____

"It is not good for the man to be alone"

—Genesis 2:18

God built into the human framework a need for intimate, honest, and warm connections with others. Relationships are a parallel—and an echo—of the relationship that God desires to have with us. (See Genesis 1:26-27.) Through good relationships, we learn more about God and how He loves us. Unfortunately, because our personal relationships are between flawed human beings, we aren't as faithful and devoted as we should be. The result is broken relationships. Let's be honest—broken relationships hurt. Even if we adopt a casual attitude and say we don't care, wrecked friendships damage and bruise.

Using the list below circle three people that represent broken relationships in your life. Perhaps it is a family member that you no longer see or talk to. Perhaps a friend who betrayed you in some way. Perhaps a business partner who didn't act in a fair and conscientious way. Perhaps a pastor who wasn't honest or moral.

Father	Mother	Boy Friend	Girl Friend
Brother	Sister	Husband	Wife
Boss	Employer	Employee	Friend
Acquaintance	Aunt	Uncle	Best Friend
Pastor	Minister	Doctor	In-law
Lawyer	Childhood Friend	Police	Teacher
Other	Other	Other	Other
_____	_____	_____	_____

Describe one of the relationships you have circled and explain the situation that broke the relationship

_____

_____

_____

_____

_____

_____

_____

How long since you had a conversation with that person and what was said in that last conversation?

_____

_____

_____

_____

_____

_____

_____

How would you describe your feelings about the broken relationship?

Resentful	Forgiving	Loathing	I don't care
Agonizing	Relief	Can't stop the pain	Longing for reconnection
Disgust	Pain	Glad it's over	Unforgiveable

Shattered relationships attack our personal self-esteem and identity. God never meant for us to feel rejected, discarded, or deserted. When these feelings are connected to the loss of a camaraderie or closeness with friends or family, we react in numerous unhealthy ways. Review the reactions below and check which symptoms describe you.

- O I wonder if that person ever thinks of me and if they hate me.

- O I refuse to get close to anyone again because I can't bear the pain.

- O I stretch the truth when telling of the incident so that I will look good.

- O I feel all alone and miserable.

- O I blame God.

- O I bake and cook and throw a party so that I will feel better or so that people will like me better.

- O I'll never admit I was wrong.

When the basic human need for connection malfunctions, we search for a replacement. Some might choose drugs, alcohol, or acting out, but we often choose food. Even when we think we have beaten that urge to eat for comfort, food is the closest substitute for the warm feeling of friendship. Health experts say that overeating is not a measure of willpower or strength or discipline, but is a direct response of our need for connection and belonging.

How does the pain of the broken relationship or rejection affect your eating habits? Be specific and honest about this aspect of your actions regarding the broken relationship or rejection.

_____

_____

_____

_____

_____

_____

_____

Rejection and broken hearts may follow us around and cause us to feel rejected even when none is intended. Such as when a friend doesn't answer your text immediately or says they can't go to the movie with you. If you feel rejected at the slightest sign, you may be over-reacting. Sometimes, no offense is intended; people are busy or distracted. Take the following True/False quiz to determine if you are overly sensitive about rejection.

○ **True** ○ **False**	If someone rejects my love, it means I am a bad person.
○ **True** ○ **False**	If someone says no to what I was trying to get them to say yes to, it means there is no good in me and I'm not important to them or I don't matter and my perspective is invalid.

O **True**	O **False**	If I want someone to like me, I must do everything they say to do.
O **True**	O **False**	If I try my best, no one will reject me.

The answer to each of these questions is false. Rejection by someone else—college entrance board, coach, friend, spouse, church committee, employer—does not define you. If you spend your life focused on what others have said or done, you will behave in response to that rejection.

Perhaps we've been conditioned since childhood to feel rejection. Let's examine our childhood.

Describe your father. Write about his personality type, his strengths and flaws, his voice, and his faith.

_____

_____

_____

_____

_____

_____

_____

_____

Consider how his actions, disposition, and temperament (or his absence) affected you.

As a small child, did you feel accepted and treasured, or rejected?

_____

_____

_____

_____

_____

How did you feel as a teenager?

_____

_____

_____

_____

_____

How did you react? (overeating, binge eating, purging, anorexia, rebellion, chose wrong crowd, promiscuity, bad attitude, etc.)

_____

_____

_____

_____

_____

Since you are now an adult, do you understand any of his actions? (such as his stresses, illnesses, pressures . . .)

_____

_____

_____

_____

_____

Describe your mother. Write about her personality type, her strengths and flaws, her voice, and her faith.

_____

_____

_____

_____

_____

Consider how her actions, disposition, and temperament (or her absence) affected you.

As a small child, did you feel accepted and treasured, or rejected?

_____

_____

_____

_____

_____

How did you feel as a teenager?

_____

_____

_____

_____

_____

How did you react? (overeating, binge eating, purging, anorexia, rebellion, chose wrong crowd, promiscuity, bad attitude, etc.)

_____

_____

_____

_____

_____

Since you are now an adult, do you understand any of her actions (such as her stresses, illnesses, pressures)?

_____

_____

_____

_____

_____

Our behaviors as children (often because we only got attention when we mis-behaved) carry over into our adult years. We may cope with rejection by eating comfort foods or by overeating, which is a conditioned response to the anger we feel. We may not even know we are angry, but we feel better when we eat.

Name a time when you were not hungry but ate anyway. Think carefully to determine what triggered that eating episode; then describe the situation here.

_____

_____

_____

_____

_____

With messages are both verbal and nonverbal, intentional and unintentional, most of us have been rejected or told we are inferior. God has called you to a great potential, not a miserable life feeling rejected. Peter gave us the plan for overcoming rejection, "So humble yourselves under the mighty power of God, and at the right time, he will lift you up in honor. Give all your worries and cares to God, for he cares about you" (1 Peter 5:6-7 NLT). Can you turn the rejection over to God and let Him deal with the person or situation? If not, why not? What is your struggle to believe what God says about you instead of the lies in your head or the lies others have told you?

_____

_____

_____

_____

_____

Forgive

It is in your best interest to forgive the person involved in your broken relationship. It isn't about him or her or whether he or she has asked for forgiveness or even whether he or she deserves to be forgiven. Instead, it is a command from God to forgive (see Mark 11:25; Luke 6:37). You will never be free from the pain until you, through an act of your will, forgive.

If forgiving is difficult for you, begin by asking God to help you become willing to forgive. Ask Him for a heart change so that, instead of feeling bitter or wanting revenge, you might be able to bless the person who hurt you. There is no room for condemnation or punishment in a forgiving heart. What is the best that could happen to them? Coming to Christ? A new job? An expanded ministry? A wonderful marriage partner? In the space below, write a prayer of blessing for that person.

_____

_____

_____

_____

_____

Yes, asking God to bless that person who hurt you is challenging, even grueling, but the result is freedom. You will be set free! It's hard to believe, but the one hurt the most by your resentment and continued bitterness is not the one who rejected you. It's you. By not moving through your hurt and anger, you are damaging your physical health, your emotions, your current relationships, and your spiritual life. God has so much more for you than being stuck in the prison of unforgiveness.

Another step you can take in forgiveness is to forgive yourself for your part in the broken relationship. Include the unhealthy choices you've made because of the failed relationship. By forgiving yourself, you will win victory over the pain and your reaction to it. For example, "I was wrong when I screamed at him, and eating cookies doesn't numb the pain. I will admit I was wrong, and I will eat when I am hungry instead of when I am angry or hurt."

If you still find forgiveness difficult and overwhelming, try to forgive by percentages. Could you make the choice to forgive him or her one percent today?[6] Write a sentence or two in the space below declaring your decision to forgive at least one percent today.

_____

_____

_____

_____

_____

Wabi Sabi

The Japanese practice of *Wabi-sabi* gives us a clue about how to handle broken relationships. When a valued vase or pitcher is broken, my inclination would be to try to glue it back together so that no one would know that it was broken. But the notion of *Wabi-sabi* handles a break differently. When a vase or dish is broken, they glue it back together with bright gold glue so that the break is noticeable. Why? Because they know that there is beauty in imperfection. Whatever pain or loss you feel only makes you a stronger, savvier, more beautiful person. In the space below, write about how your broken relationship has changed you for the better and how you will handle relationships in the future.

_____

_____

_____

_____

_____

_____

_____

_____

_____

Two New Relationships

First, Jesus Christ. You will go through lonely times in life, but you'll never go through it alone if you have an intimate relationship with Jesus Christ. A relationship with Him is worth 10,000 human relationships. He will never forsake you or hurt you. Begin now to renew your personal daily time of reading the Bible and praying. Put your devotional time on your schedule. Read slowly, considering each word. Relational reading of the Bible means applying the promises and truth to your personal situation. Insert your name into the Scripture as you read. Write a verse on a card and read it all through the day. Write a prayer in the space below. First express your love for God and then ask Him to show you how to develop a closer relationship with Him.

_____

_____

_____

_____

_____

_____

_____

Second, new friends. Make new relationships by committing to being a friend. Think of some of the qualities of a good friend, and then seek to be that kind of person. "The world is full of people waiting to be loved. Stop saying, 'I don't have any friends!' and start saying, 'God, who can you use me to minister to? Who can I show your love to?'"[7] In the space below, make a list of ways that you can become a better friend to others. Then write a short prayer asking God to help you develop strong, loyal friendships.

_____

_____

_____

_____

_____

_____

_____

_____

_____

_____

_____

_____

_____

_____

_____

CHAPTER FIVE: REMEMBERING LOST DREAMS

"Life's funny. You have to find a way to keep going, to keep laughing, even after you realize that none of your dreams will come true. When you realize that, there's still so much of a life to get through."[8]

Look back a few years or longer and remember a dream you had as a child, a teen, or a younger adult. Write a few sentences about that dream here.

_____

_____

_____

_____

_____

_____

Did the dream come true? If yes, how? If no, why not?

_____

_____

_____

_____

_____

_____

_____

If your dream came true, how did it make you feel?

○   I felt happy and fulfilled.

○   It wasn't what I thought it would be.

○   No one seemed to care about my feelings.

If you haven't accomplished that dream yet, how do you feel about it?

○   I'm discouraged.

○   I feel defeated.

○   I'm mad at myself.

○   I'm angry with someone else.

○   It is too late now.

Our dreams and plans are a combination of our experiences, personality, abilities, passions, and motivations. Evaluate your background, including your family, education, previous jobs, travels, and events, and then describe how your experiences have influenced your dream.

_____

_____

_____

_____

_____

_____

Have your experiences made you

Wise	Mature	Cynical
Mean	Joyful	Unstable
Funny	Stable	Unwilling to commit
Clingy	Irresponsible	Responsible
Sad	Shrewd	Hard to live with
Pleasant	Perceptive	Insightful
Cunning	Other_____	Other_____

Our natural abilities and talents also contribute to the dreams we dream. It's been said that the average person is endowed with more than 700 skills. You may be a gifted musician or artist. You may have been born with a knack for words and have the gift of gab. You may be a natural athlete or have an easy competence for math. Next to each of the words below, name one of your gifts. Each of us has gifts that we don't notice or that we feel embarrassed to mention, but we encourage you to work hard to name at least one gift for each word and not leave any blanks. If you are stuck, ask a friend.

Talent _____

Flair_____

Skill_____

Knack _____

Potential _____

Ability _____

Another contributor to our dreams is passion. Our passions are made up of desires, hopes, and ambitions.

What do you love to do?

_____

_____

_____

_____

_____

_____

What interests and excites you?

_____

_____

_____

_____

_____

_____

_____

What do you care about?

_____

_____

_____

_____

_____

_____

_____

_____

_____

_____

You are a package deal. All your experiences, talents, abilities, and passions wrapped up together are what make you able to dream big dreams.

Below are some common reactions to the destruction of a dream:

Apathy (why try?)	Give up	Work harder	Denial
Change my attitude	Eat sweets	Isolation	Crying
Fear	Anxiety	Shame	Overeat
Quiet	Realistic	Hopeful	Thrifty

How has the realization of that dream or the loss of that dream affected your eating habits?

Do you eat when you feel depressed about the dream? Explain.

_____

_____

_____

Do you eat when you are happy about the dream? Explain.

_____

_____

_____

Did your eating habits play a role in the loss of the dream? Explain.

_____

_____

_____

_____

Why do you think eating has a relationship to that dream? Explain.

_____

_____

_____

_____

God's Dream for Abram

God said, "Look up at the sky and count the stars—if indeed you can count them"

—Genesis 15:5, NIV

God promised Abram descendants so plentiful that they could not be numbered. Yet for years, nothing happened, and Abram's wife, Sarai, didn't have even one child. How could the promise be true? So Abram tried to figure out a human way. God could keep the promise if Abram's servant Eliezer became the heir to carry on the family name.

But God took Abram outside and showed him the stars in the sky and said, "Look up! I am still God and your dream is in my hands" (paraphrased). The next verse (Genesis 15:6) shows Abram's reaction: "Abram believed the Lord."

Whatever your dream, God's dream is bigger. Write a commitment in the space below declaring that you are willing to believe God in the same way Abram believed. If you're not ready to make a commitment, what's holding you back?

"No eye has seen, no ear has heard, and no mind has imagined what God has prepared for those who love him" (1 Corinthians 2:9, NLT). Do you believe God like Abram did? If not, why not?

_____

_____

_____

_____

_____

_____

_____

Grieve

Whether a result of a broken relationship, missed opportunity, poor choice, or difficult childhood, the fact is, all losses need to be grieved.[9]

When you think about the loss of your dream, do you ask yourself these questions?

- What did I do wrong?

- Could I have done anything differently?

- If only I hadn't _____ .

- If only I had _____ .

Why do you think these are the wrong questions to ask?

_____

_____

_____

_____

_____

_____

_____

_____

_____

_____

If your dream is delayed, broken, or lost, can you believe God (as Abram did in Genesis 15:10)? Write a prayer expressing your sorrow about the dream that seems lost. Tell God you are willing to let the dream go if that is His plan. Tell Him you are also willing to wait.

_____

_____

_____

_____

_____

_____

_____

_____

_____

It is never too late. The movie producer Steven Spielberg was rejected from film school three times. The manager of the Grand Ole Opry told Elvis Presley he should go back to driving a truck. A newspaper editor fired Walt Disney because he "lacked imagination." Even if your situation seems impossible, or you think you have made too many mistakes, the dream—if it is God's dream—can come true. Don't turn to food to comfort you for the loss; turn to Jesus.

How can you change your actions to reflect your new belief that God is able? What will you do about each of these situations?

Eating sweets: _____

_____

Snacking: _____

_____

Binge eating: _____

_____

My view of God: _____

_____

Sticking with FP4H: _____

_____

Believing in the dream: _____

_____

CHAPTER SIX: UNDERSTANDING PERSONALITY

Take or retake the Linked© Personality Assessment in Appendix One at the back of this book.

List your scores for each personality type here:

Mobilizer _____

Socializer _____

Organizer_____

Stabilizer _____

Circle your personality combination (the dominant personality—highest score—listed first)

Mobilizer/Socializer	Organizer/Mobilizer
Mobilizer/Organizer	Organizer/Stabilizer
Socializer/Mobilizer	Stabilizer/Socializer
Socializer/Stabilizer	Stabilizer/Organizer

If your top two scores show any combination other than those listed above, you may be checking some attributes that are learned behavior instead of instinctive personality traits. We suggest that you answer each line again in a different colored ink and then total all the scores. It is possible to camouflage your true personality if you have a life situation or a career that compels you to fit into a compensation mold. For example, a pastor's wife often scores evenly on all four personality types because, in her position, she is often called upon to be all things to all people. By completing the profile a second time and combining the scores, the underlying personality traits will surface.

1. List three personality traits that you checked in the weaknesses of your primary personality type.

    a. _____

    b. _____

    c. _____

2. List three personality traits that you checked in the weaknesses of your secondary personality type.

    a. _____

    b. _____

    c. _____

As you review these six personality traits listed above, consider the limitations that each one places on your life in general and on your ability to get to your health and wellness goals. List some of those limitations below.

1. _____

    _____

    _____

2. _____

_____

_____

3. _____

_____

_____

4. _____

_____

_____

5. _____

_____

6. _____

_____

_____

Now carefully review the six traits you listed above and honestly evaluate which of these traits produces selfishness in you. For example, a socializer personality weakness is "wanting attention," which might lead to manipulation of others to get noticed. A stabilizer personality weakness is "procrastination," which he uses to control others. A mobilizer personality weakness is "power," in which she may do anything to obtain authority. A organizer personality weakness is "moodiness," where she may use moods to get her way.

List each of your six weaker traits again and write a sentence honestly assessing how you use this trait to get your way.

1. _____
   _____
   _____

2. _____
   _____
   _____

3. _____
   _____
   _____

4. _____
   _____
   _____

5. _____
   _____

6. _____
   _____
   _____

Understanding your personality and its relationship to selfishness may open up some new ways to look at how selfishness affects your eating habits.

Select the best answer

Because I often feel I am right and no one listens, I

○ grab a sugary snack to make me feel better.

○ start cooking the favorite foods of others so that they will have good thoughts about me.

○ go through the drive-thru window at a fast food place and tell no one what I ate or drank.

○ Other _____

_____

My house is a mess and there is too much to do, so I

○ search for a salty or creamy treat to eat while sitting in front of the TV.

○ stand at the pantry or refrigerator door and search for anything to eat.

○ search the internet for new and interesting recipes.

○ Other _____

_____

Everyone seems to want me to do something for them and I feel overwhelmed, so I

○   find a mindless TV show or surf the internet to get away from them.

○   bury myself in a page-turning novel.

○   complain about the inconvenience while eating cake.

○   Other _____

       _____

Personality traits are built into your temperament. Operating in the strengths of your personality type will bring fulfillment and balance unless you allow your strengths to overpower you. When this happens, the strengths become obsessions or weaknesses. Any strength carried to its extreme becomes a weakness.

For example, a mobilizer who is a strong, decisive person capable of making good choices (a strength) can become a know-it-all who thinks he or she is never wrong and demands that everyone do what he or she says. The ability to make good choices becomes a blind spot that makes you believe you are more capable than anyone else and therefore your choices should rule. If you are a mobilizer personality, how can you temper this good trait so that you do not become domineering and demanding? If you know someone or live with someone who is a mobilizer personality, how can you cope with their outbursts without turning to food?

_____

_____

_____

_____

_____

One of the strengths of a organizer personality is order and excellence. But taken to the extreme, this good trait becomes obsession and the person becomes trapped in the grip of perfectionism—consumed with organizing sock drawers and alphabetizing spice racks, demanding that everyone else also be perfect and on time. If you are a organizer personality, how can you temper this good trait so that you do not become fixated and consumed by order? If you know someone or live with someone who is a organizer personality, how can you cope with his or her fanaticism without turning to food?

_____

_____

_____

_____

_____

A socializer just wants to have fun, but taken to the extreme, this delightful and positive trait becomes a ruse to shirk responsibility—or as an excuse to go shopping, causing financial problems. If you are a socializer personality, how can you temper this good trait so that you are reliable as well as playful? If you know someone or live with someone who is a socializer personality, how can you cope with their humorous and mischievous behavior without turning to food?

_____

_____

_____

_____

_____

_____

A stabilizer personality wants peace and calm, but that tranquility can become procrastination, compromising standards, and blocking out real feelings if he or she is goaded. If you are a stabilizer personality, how can you temper this good trait so that you are not only relaxed but also successful at work and relationships? If you know someone or live with someone who is a stabilizer personality, how can you cope with his or her laid-back behavior without turning to food?

———————————————————————————————

———————————————————————————————

———————————————————————————————

———————————————————————————————

———————————————————————————————

Personality traits lived in the extreme may play a large role in eating disorders and poor eating habits. Living in your weaknesses can lead to anxious behavior and depression, which then lead to difficulty managing your weight and eating healthily. Researchers Carmen Keller and Michael Siegrist, who published their findings in the *Journal of American College Health*, revealed that a person's personality determines why and what he or she eats. For example, "A lack of conscientiousness leads people to eat impulsively and to lose self-control in the face of tempting food situations with palatable and nicely smelling and tasting food. Neurotic people may eat too much high-caloric food to deal with their negative emotions."[10] The study revealed that those who are more social and extroverted, like the socializer and mobilizer personalities, tend to associate fun with food. In contrast, personality traits such as perfectionism play into the reasons for anorexia, bulimia, or binge eating. We compare ourselves to others, judging unrealistically that if we were thinner, we would be better liked and more successful—so we go on a fad diet or starve ourselves. Or we take the opposite, more arrogant approach: we binge-eat without caring about calories or nutrition.

Which of your personality traits do you like best?

_____

_____

_____

_____

_____

When you are in that moment or exhibiting that personality trait, pay attention to how it affects your eating:

O I like myself so much at that moment that I eat anything I want to eat in any quantity I want.

O I love the feeling so much that I feel in control and make good food choices.

O Other _____

_____

Which of your personality traits do you like the least?

_____

_____

_____

_____

_____

When you are in that moment or exhibiting that personality trait, pay attention to how it affects your eating:

○ I hate myself so much at that moment that I eat anything I want to eat in any quantity I want.

○ I hate that feeling so much that I decide to make changes and act differently, including my food choices.

○ Other _____

_____

Read the sentence below:

Using food as a reward for my behavior and personality is a good way to live in my strengths.

Is this sentence true or false?

Why?

_____

_____

_____

_____

_____

_____

_____

_____

CHAPTER SEVEN: IDENTIFYING SELFISHNESS

One of the first bits of truth we must discover about ourselves is that we are naturally selfish. It's part of being human. Understanding our self-seeking, self-interested nature is critical to preventing our ego from sabotaging our wellness.

Review these selfish traits. Check all that apply.

○   I want to impress people.

○   I always think of myself first.

○   I love stuff.

○   I deserve the best.

○   I don't care.

○   I want to be first.

○   I just want _____

How do these traits affect your eating habits?

○   I hide snacks so that there will be enough for me.

○   I am impatient when meals take too long to prepare, so I snack and graze.

○   I make non-conscious food choices.

○   I give in to poor food choices, because I deserve to feel happy.

○   When I'm too busy, I eat unhealthy snacks.

○   I don't tell the whole truth when I complete my food tracker.

○   When I'm unhappy, eating brings me comfort.

Disorders, such as anorexia and bulimia, may need medical care. Disordered eating may be due to a selfish attitude such as, "I want what I want. I want to be thin and in control of what I eat no matter the consequence." Overeating does not make us more selfish than other people, but the compulsion to have what we want when we want it can contribute to overeating. There is a fine line between taking care of self and excessive self-concern or self-soothing strategies that turn into full-blown selfishness.

Read these Bible verses about selfishness:

Don't be selfish; don't try to impress others. Be humble, thinking of others as better than yourselves
—Philippians 2:3 (NLT)

For jealousy and selfishness are not God's kind of wisdom
—James 3:15 (NLT)

But David said, "No, my brothers! Don't be selfish with what the LORD has given us. He has kept us safe and helped us defeat the band of raiders that attacked us"
—1 Samuel 30:23 (NLT)

Then Jesus said to his disciples, "If any of you wants to be my follower, you must turn from your selfish ways, take up your cross, and follow me"
—Matthew 16:24 (NLT)

Don't be concerned for your own good but for the good of others

—1 Corinthians 10:24 (NLT)

If someone has enough money to live well and sees a brother or sister in need but shows no compassion—how can God's love be in that person?

—1 John 3:17 (NLT)

For each selfish attitude or trait below, draw a line to God's solution (using the answers found in the verses quoted above).

Selfish	Take up your cross
Trying to impress	Show compassion
Jealousy	Humble yourself
Ego	Think of others first
Pride	God's wisdom
Hoarding	Recognize God's provision

Using the list in the left column, identify two attitudes that portray your feelings most of the time.

1. _____

2. _____

Write a sentence about these two attitudes describing how each one affects your eating habits. You'll need to think carefully to uncover the effect of this connection. Thoroughly take inventory of your thoughts, attitudes, and viewpoints. Honestly facing a selfish mindset is the only way to destroy it.

1. _____

_____

_____

2. _____

_____

_____

Beyond Selfishness

A sense of self and true identity is critical to wellness. As believers, our identity is not found in our looks, our weight, or what others think of us. Our identity is found in Jesus only. We are His masterpiece and the object of His love. Allowing true identity to warp into self obsession is never God's plan for us.

Selfishness builds walls. We withdraw from others by shutting down and refusing to talk. Or we create an impenetrable barrier between us and the person. Or we seek comfort from food. Or we pretend not to care and become superficial. How do you protect yourself when faced with

Ridicule? _____

_____

Shame? _____

_____

Insult? _____

_____

Indifference? _____

_____

Other? _____

_____

Now consider how to respond to these situations without self-protection—knowing that you are the precious child of God and your identity is in Him, not in the opinion of others. Write what you think Jesus would do when faced with

Ridicule? _____

_____

Shame? _____

_____

Insult? _____

_____

Indifference? _____

_____

Other? _____

_____

Another way to move beyond selfishness is a determined effort to be vulnerable with honesty and courage.

Using the list below, write what you'd like to share with a trusted friend about each subject.

Hopes _____

_____

Fears _____

_____

Desires _____

_____

Dislikes _____

_____

Feelings _____

_____

Thoughts _____

_____

What is keeping you from sharing these deep ideas with someone?

_____

_____

_____

_____

_____

Do you have a friend who is trustworthy? On the list below, circle the characteristics that you most value in a trustworthy friend.

Loyal	Fair	Honest
Caring	Loving	Non-judging
Positive	Listener	Wise

Share deeply personal information with a trustworthy friend. Stand tall, make good eye contact, and tell the truth. It is a relationship risk, but the connection with another person will catapult you from selfishness to kindness and a generous spirit. From self-serving to self-disclosure is a big leap but well worth it.

God Focus

God has made it clear that He wants us to know Him intimately. If we are focused on ourselves, we will not comprehend or appreciate His love, grace, and mercy. His love is unconditional. He loves us with no prerequisites. In the space below, make a list of ways that you recognize God's love for you.

_____

_____

_____

_____

Caring for Others

We were made to care about others—not to be self-centered—and to love others with unconditional love. No requirements, no restrictions, no preconditions. Changing our focus from self to others will help us move beyond selfishness. However, if you are in a destructive relationship, you must set boundaries to protect yourself. If you are in that situation, consider talking to a pastor or health-care professional.

> *"If selfishness is the key to being miserable, then selflessness must be the key to being happy!"*
>
> ~Joyce Meyer

Write how you feel about changing your focus from self to others. Be honest with yourself.

_____

_____

_____

_____

Ask God to reveal any behavior (especially related to eating) that is rooted in self-centeredness. Write a few sentences about what He brings to light for you.

_____

_____

_____

_____

_____

In the space below, write a prayer asking God to remove self-seeking and self-interest from your heart.

_____

_____

_____

_____

_____

_____

_____

CHAPTER EIGHT: EXPOSING ANGER

Anger is the source of many of our difficulties. Yet we may not know that we are angry. We think we feel calm and relaxed in times of confusion or lack of concentration, but the foundation of these issues is often anger. Even physical symptoms, such as headache and asthma episodes, may stem from an irritation or fury within. Our reaction is negative behavior, such as temper loss, rage, insomnia, neglecting responsibilities, and overeating.

Healthy and Unhealthy Anger Scale

Healthy	Mild	Serious	Extreme
Frustrated	Ticked Off	Irritated	Enraged

In fact, anger is a common trigger for overeating. Overeating is not always a lack of willpower or discipline. We are not really lazy or weak because we eat too much. Anger may be the issue that causes us to eat more than we need.

Name three situations where you feel angry. (Consider your typical week's agenda, your commute to work, the people in your life, the lack of resources, the demands made on you, your personal space, etc.)

1. _____

_____

2. _____

_____

3. _____

_____

Describe how you calm yourself when you face these situations.

1. _____

_____

2. _____

_____

3. _____

_____

Anger may flare up when we are faced with other trigger emotions. In the list below, circle emotions that you often feel.

Misunderstood	Exasperated	Lost
Fearful	Provoked	Isolated
Frustrated	Irritated	Annoyed
Rejected	Infuriated	Dissatisfied
Disappointed	Busy	Bothered

For each of the emotions that you circled, describe why you feel that way. For example, "I am so busy because it seems I must do everything for everyone in my family. I cook, clean, do the laundry, monitor the homework, run a taxi service for my kids. I wish I had some down time or could at least slow down."

_____

_____

_____

_____

_____

_____

Review the three anger situations you listed and assign to each one an under-lying emotion from the list above. For example, "When someone at church or school asks me to take on a responsibility, I bristle because I already have so much to do. Can't they see that I am a busy woman?"

_____

_____

_____

_____

_____

_____

Now let's consider what is happening in the brain when anger rises up. Scientists say that more than 10,000 chemical reactions happen every second in the brain, responding to what we see, hear, touch, smell, taste, and feel. The signals from our senses alert the brain, which tells our body what to do. We may calm down because a situation is in control, or we may snap into action because there is danger. When the signal is stressful and anger inducing, we often turn to food. In fact, anger is the best path to food binges—not one cookie, but a dozen or the whole package.[11]

True hunger isn't affected by anger, but eating and overeating episodes are fre-quently a result of anger. Next to each of the following situations, list a type of anger (rage, seething, irritation, annoyance, sulkiness, shouting, revenge, etc.) you feel and then name a food you would love to eat in that situation.

Anger Situation	Type of Anger	Food I'd Like to Eat
Stress at work		
Dangerous drivers on the road		
Fight with spouse		
Teenager attitudes		
Hurtful words from a friend		
Job loss		
Financial stress		
Physical pain		

We tend to think of food in anger situations because our brains are built to quickly react with a soothing solution—sometimes with the quickest, easiest way to pleasure, which is food. When someone cuts us off on the freeway, our brain says, *Go through the fast-food drive-in.* Perhaps some of your food choices were childhood favorites, or you love the aroma or the creaminess or the crunch. Something in your brain seeks the pleasure and satisfaction of that particular food—counteracting the anger tantrum deep inside. Why do you think that willpower is no match for this powerful brain function?

_____

_____

_____

_____

Owning the Anger

Turning to food when anger rages is often about not wanting to feel the anger. Stuffing food stuffs anger, but it doesn't avoid anger.

Facing anger with food is only a temporary fix. When we have eaten all we can hold, the anger will still be there and so will the weight gain from the food. Now we can add anger at ourselves to the anger over the situation. We need to understand and embrace the feeling of anger—to recognize the anger and feel it. Feeling the anger doesn't mean that we must express it, especially negatively or in the moment of its greatest intensity.

What person are you angry with? (self, a person from your past, a boss, a spouse, a friend, a pastor, etc.)

_____

_____

_____

_____

What situation are you angry about? (job, marriage, family, church, etc.)

_____

_____

_____

_____

_____

If we can own our anger by recognizing it and facing it and feeling it, then we can defeat this enemy of our soul, which affects our weight and health.

Begin by recognizing and accepting the angry undertones in your behavior. From the exercises above, what do you believe is your greatest anger trigger?

_____

_____

_____

_____

_____

Changing anger patterns is not an instantaneous fix. Becoming aware of why you feel anger is the crucial first step. Then, it will take time and repeated effort. God said to deal with anger issues each day before we go to bed. "Be angry and do not sin; do not let the sun go down on your anger, and give no opportunity to the devil" (Ephesians 4:26-27, ESV). In the space below, describe your nighttime routine from when you decide to go to bed until you fall asleep. For example,

"Prepare a glass of ice water for my bedside table, brush my teeth, wash my face, change into fresh pajamas, pull the covers down, put lotion on my hands, write in my journal, read a chapter from the Bible, pray, turn out the lights."

_____

_____

_____

_____

_____

Now add a new step into your routine. Think back over your day. Identify any person or situation that triggered your anger today. Remember that nobody causes our feelings. Our feelings are ours. But certain situations may trigger angry feelings. Name it and feel it. Now ask God to help you defeat it.

_____

_____

_____

_____

Some of us may need to change our reaction time in order to overcome anger. The Bible says, "Know this, my beloved brothers: let every person be quick to hear, slow to speak, slow to anger; for the anger of man does not produce the righteousness of God" (James 1:19-20, ESV). The following are some suggestions about how to slow down your anger reaction time. Which idea can you implement? Add other ideas that will help you apply the brakes to your anger.

- ○ Count to 10 or 100.

- ○ Breathe. (Investigate the exercises you can do to calm yourself through breathing.)

- Take a walk.

- Walk away from the person without saying a word.

- Say James 1:19-20 aloud.

_____

_____

_____

_____

_____

Anger does not have to be a regular part of our lives. We can do something about it by admitting that we are angry. Only then can we be healed. Only then can we stop the cycle of anger and overeating. Removing anger will allow good emotions to surface and will leave room for love and joy and creativity to emerge.

CHAPTER NINE: UNCOVERING NEGATIVITY

You have met her, haven't you? That girl who sees the bad side of every situation and predicts gloom and doom. She is so consumed by the bad, she can't see the good. Negativity is all around us, and the people who are negative drain us, emotionally and physically

Who is the most negative person you know?

_____

_____

_____

_____

_____

_____

What does this person do or say that is negative?

_____

_____

_____

_____

_____

What kind of atmosphere does the negativity produce? Circle all that apply.

Contradictions   Disagreements   Pessimism

Gloom   Hostility   Criticism

Blame   Rebellion   Denial

Opposition   Dissatisfaction   Discouragement

When reacting to the negativity and the atmosphere it produces, describe how you respond:

O   Physically: eating or starving?

O   Mentally: arguing or ignoring?

O   Emotionally: tears or anger?

O   Spiritually: prayer or rebuke?

When others are negative, do you . . .

O   take it personally, assuming you did something wrong?

O   beg the person to see the positive side?

O   find a comforting food to help you face it or cope with it?

Negative people are typically negative about many parts of their life, so their misery is not about you. You can protect yourself by spending time with positive people and by pursuing activities that make you happy, such as sports, dancing, hobbies, and church. But the relief from the negative words of others is not found in the pantry or refrigerator.

Be a Negativity Killer

You can be free from negativity by choosing your attitude and response. You may not be able to change the negative person, but you can refuse to feed his or her pessimism. Instead of quarreling or disagreeing, say a kind word. Tell the person you love them. Give them a hug. Kindness is a negativity killer. When faced with an unpleasant person, such as a waiter or store clerk, say thank you, bless him or her with a big tip, look him or her in the eye, and smile.

This week, look for an opportunity to be a negativity killer. Report the event back to your class by writing about it here.

_____

_____

_____

_____

Negativity in Myself

Negativity shows up in our thoughts and conversations too. In fact, in the amygdala region of the brain, which regulates emotions and motivation, about two-thirds of this brain section is to detect bad news. That only leaves one-third of the region for good news. No wonder we seek delicious, creamy, sweet, satisfying food—we are seeking good and avoiding bad.

Typically, when we are stressed and overcommitted or we have failed to accomplish our goals, negativity creeps in. Winning the battle against negativity requires some internal changes and some deliberate actions, beginning with attitude.

Attitude

Changing my attitude requires intentional removal of unhelpful thoughts and pessimism. When faced with the damage of a windstorm, I felt overwhelmed and paralyzed. And I said so—often. "What will we do?" "There's too much work." FP4H director emeritus Carole Lewis calls these kinds of thoughts *stinkin' thinkin'*.

What are some stinkin' thinkin' thoughts that come into your mind?

When a friend doesn't call _____

_____

When someone else gets the promotion _____

_____

When hurtful words are said _____

_____

When you've eaten too much _____

_____

When you can't get into that pair of pants you wore last week _____

_____

When trouble strikes you unexpectedly _____

_____

One morning after a windstorm, my daughter reminded me to change my attitude by changing my words. I began to speak positively. "We have a plan." "The cleanup will begin today." "We will come out on the other side." And I began to get stronger and healthier. When my attitude is doom and gloom, my brain thinks, *Food will make me feel better.* But a change of attitude is much better than food.

Name a time when your attitude caused you to seek food for comfort.

_____

_____

_____

_____

You can eliminate this kind of stinkin' thinkin' in the future by the words you speak to yourself. In the space below, write three sentences that are positive and uplifting. Use this self-talk instead of negativity.

1. _____

_____

2. _____

_____

3. _____

_____

The second powerful tool to use against negativity is gratitude. The Bible counsels us to "give thanks for everything" (Ephesians 5:20, NLT). When we are thankful, we are not whining. Be honest as you think about your problems. Isn't there a good side? If you were involved in an accident and the car is totaled, what is the good side? No one was hurt? If someone was hurt, is there a good side? The rescue team got them to the hospital. If your home was damaged in a storm or flood, what good can you find? A beloved animal survived? You were safe? Even in the worst circumstances, such as great loss and pain and death, there is always a blessing to be found—if you look for it.

Do these situations drive you to the refrigerator? Describe how it happens.

_____

_____

_____

Gratitude is the answer to that burning pain of heartache. Begin with a small blank notebook and start a thankful list. Make it your goal to write a thankful sentence for a person, object, or situation at least once each day. Try to reach 1,000 thankful entries. It will take months and months to reach 1,000, but you will develop the gratitude habit.

Begin here with the first three entries you will put into your notebook.

1. _____

   _____

2. _____

   _____

3. _____

   _____

The third powerful tool for overcoming negativity is to focus on servanthood instead of self. Most of our complaints center on ourselves.

- Why didn't I get the _____? (job, part, guy, . . .)

- She didn't _____me. (call, invite, include, . . .)

- What they said hurt my feelings because _____

When we change the focus from ourselves to others, our negativity (and the pain and misery it brings) begins to disappear.

There are numerous ways you can bless and serve others. For example, in a restaurant, treat the wait staff with kindness by saying thank you. Look them in the eye when they refill your glass or cup; acknowledge the service with thoughtful words. Pay the meal ticket for someone else in the restaurant, but ask the waiter not to tell them who paid. Pay the toll for the car behind you. When you give a tip to the wait staff or the airport luggage handlers or anyone who has helped you, give the most generous tip possible. Walk away before they realize that you have been so generous. Say to yourself, "I blessed someone today for Jesus' sake." Notice how you feel after you have acted selflessly and generously.

When you focus on others with a servant's heart and a goal to bless them, you will defeat negativity.

CHAPTER TEN: RECOGNIZING RESENTMENTS

"The word resentment comes from the Latin word *sentire* which means, 'to feel,' and when you put 're' in front of any word, it means 'again,' so the word resentment means 'to feel again.'"[12]

Life is full of situations that can feel like neglect and injury. We react to those mistreatments by holding a grudge. If harbored long enough, that grudge becomes bitterness and hatred. And when we share these feelings with friends, we receive encouragement that we were right and justified in the situation, so we hold the grudge longer, and it grows into resentment.

Resentment damages us profoundly. Alice May said, "Hanging on to a resentment is like drinking poison and hoping it will kill someone else."[13] Resentments festering in us become entrenched and rooted until we are exhausted from carrying them around. Frederick Nietzche said, "Nothing on earth consumes a man more quickly than the passion of resentment."

Many of us would say we don't resent anything and can't imagine that resentments could have anything to do with overeating or unhealthy eating; but when we look deeper, we may discover issues we didn't realize were there.

From the list below, mark food situations that are familiar to you.

○ I get angry with myself for overeating—again.

○ Why does every activity have to center around food?

○ Some friends and family push me to eat more or try a dish I shouldn't eat.

○ Why are some people so slim—my legs weren't that thin when I was 12.

○ Exercise is hard for me, but other people seem to love it.

○ I can never get motivated, no matter how good my intentions.

○ I've gained weight, but my high school friends still look slim.

○ I resent it when other people buy junk food and leave it around to tempt me.

○ Why can't I lose weight as fast as I gain it?

Now mark the life situations that cause you pain.

○ My boss rarely notices my work and someone else gets the attention or promotion.

○ Being a wife and mother is hard work, and no one helps.

○ I hate being responsible for everything.

○ I don't think I should have to do all the work around the house and pay the bills too.

○ I have to work at a job while other moms get to stay home.

○ I am stuck at home babysitting and running a taxi service for my kids when I could have a career and adult conversations every day.

○ I wish I had a best friend.

○ I wish I could talk to someone about my sex life.

○ My friend's marriage seems happy, yet my spouse and I fight almost every night.

○ My spouse's job isn't as prestigious as someone else's job.

○ My family is dysfunctional.

○ My mom and I don't get along.

○ My church doesn't seem to care about me and my problems.

A resentment begins with an offense or a situation that you cannot seem to change. Resentments can be toward family, authorities, or self. Resentments carry regret and worry around like a full backpack. We deal with resentments by blaming the world (*everyone is against me*), or by letting past hurts, insecurities, and pride control us. Review the resentments you checked in the lists above, and write about each one. How do you feel about these situations now? Has the resentment grown as time has passed? Can you think of any solution that would begin healing the resentment?

_____

_____

_____

_____

Self-resentment is one of the hardest strongholds to break, especially when it's related to our perception of our body. Using the list below, write about how you feel about these body parts.

Eyes _____

_____

Nose _____

_____

Feet _____

_____

Skin _____

_____

Height _____

_____

Weight _____

_____

Body shape _____

_____

Did you notice any bitterness or loathing in your descriptions of yourself? Self-hatred is not what God planned. David understood this when he wrote, "I praise you because I am fearfully and wonderfully made; your works are wonderful, I know that full well" (Psalm 139:14, NIV). God made us just as He intended us to look—curly hair, long nose, thin lips and all. He adores all our little quirks.

God did not intend for us to abuse and mistreat our bodies. Unfortunately, we have unhealthy habits, and we have harmed ourselves with overeating or unhealthy foods that injure our bodies. In the space below, write an honest appraisal of how you have damaged your health by poor choices.

_____

_____

_____

_____

_____

_____

_____

Resentment toward others or self can sometimes lead to poor choices in food and life. We think the resentment is acceptable and reasonable, but it is destructive. Resentment takes us nowhere positive; instead, it drags us deeper into bad decisions regarding health and lifestyle. Resentment is futile and will not change our situation. Resentments lead to jealousy, fear, frustration, dissatisfaction, and exasperation. When we wallow in the resentment, we head for the pantry or refrigerator. As long as we hold on to resentment, we will continue to move toward our next poor food choice.

Think of one person you resent or feel hostility toward. Write his or her name in the space below. Then write a note to that person describing the situation and telling him or her you will no longer let the resentment toward him or her build in your mind. You may never approach the person or allow that person to read your words, but writing them down will break the chains of resentment.

_____

_____

_____

_____

_____

_____

_____

_____

_____

_____

_____

_____

_____

Think of one organization or authority that you resent or feel hostility toward. Write the name in the space below. Then write a paragraph or so describing the situation and releasing them from responsibility for your pain. Freedom begins with confession.

_____

_____

_____

_____

_____

_____

_____

_____

_____

Now pick one resentment you have about yourself or your life. In the space below, write about it, describing your feelings. Then write a prayer asking God to help you accept what you cannot change and for His help to change your attitudes and actions regarding the difficulty.

_____

_____

_____

_____

_____

_____

_____

_____

_____

_____

CHAPTER ELEVEN: CELEBRATION

As a disciple of Jesus, our goal is to live as if we were Him, because we represent Him. Dallas Willard said that the apprenticed life is "conducting the usual activities of life—home, school, community, business, government—in the character and power of Jesus."

Peter and Paul understood walking in the path of Jesus.

Grow in the grace and knowledge of our Lord and Savior Jesus Christ

—2 Peter 3:18 (NLT)

Whether then you eat or drink or whatever you do, do all to the glory of God

—1 Corinthians 10:31 (NLT)

Review the issues we've covered in these past weeks. Remember how each one affects your eating habits. Then write what God has shown you in your personal-discovery assignment and how you will modify your eating habits and behavioral responses to this loss in the future.

Chapter Two – Acknowledging Disobedience

Chapter Three – Discovering My Assets and Flaws

Chapter Four – Exploring Rejection and Broken Relationships

Chapter Five – Remembering Lost Dreams

Chapter Six – Understanding Personality

Chapter Seven – Identifying Selfishness

Chapter Eight – Exposing Anger

Chapter Nine – Uncovering Negativity

Chapter Ten – Recognizing Resentments

We follow Him because we have confidence in Him. Our lives are attached to His life. And we place ourselves squarely on His shoulders and face every stronghold because of His strength. We will not allow loss of any possession, position, or person to push us into the cycle of overeating and weight gain. When facing your problems causes you to be disappointed and discouraged, say the words of the undaunted Christopher Columbus: "Today we sail on."

Confidence in Him takes resolve, determination, dedication, and tenacity, regardless of what happens. Today make it your goal to never give in to the pressures to mindlessly eat or to eat high-fat, high-calorie foods for comfort or to compensate for loss.

Your future health requires resolve and perseverance. The famous preacher Charles Spurgeon observed that "The snail: Through perseverance made it to the ark." Remember Paul, who was hated, stoned, jailed, and rejected. Yet he always "went to the next city."

It is always too soon to quit.

> *The key is trusting Christ. Obey Him and give Him the throne in your heart. Peter said, "...in your hearts set apart Christ as Lord"*
>
> *— 1 Peter 3:15(NLT)*

Looking into a Mirror

In a mirror, we see the flaws and mistakes—such as blood on a man's collar after shaving or lipstick on a woman's nose. The Word of God is our mirror. It tells the truth about us. What does the Word reveal to you?

- Your prayer life needs help.

- Some bitterness or resentment is lodged inside.

- Your worship is shallow.

- Your relationships are messed up.

Look carefully, closely, seriously. The mirror of God's Word is the only way to see the other side of our fears. True freedom includes the freedom to tell God things we cannot say aloud. Answer the questions below with your thoughts, including Scripture verses that apply.

Who am I?

_____

_____

_____

_____

What shapes me?

_____

_____

_____

_____

What forces do I allow to shape me?

_____

_____

_____

_____

Is God at work?

_____

_____

_____

_____

Am I willing to allow God to change my health, including my eating habits and
my exercising habits?

_____

_____

_____

_____

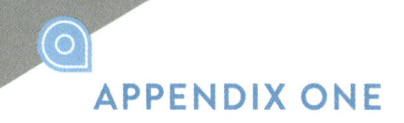

IDENTIFY YOUR PERSONALITY (WHO YOU ARE)

You may have heard about personalities for many years. Perhaps, you've never had the opportunity to know what personality you are and how it applies to your relationships. It may have never occurred to you how your personality affects your journey toward wellness. It only takes a few minutes to determine what your dominant personality is. The best way to figure it out is to take the LINKED® Personality Assessment below.

Circle the answers that best describe you. Mark only one per question. Be as honest as you can. This assessment helps you discover how you would respond in everyday situations. Don't over think. Your first response is usually the best one.

Circle the answers that describe how you react most often. Go with your first thought, be as honest as you can, and don't over think your answers. For best results, don't answer thinking, "Is this a good or bad choice?" Mark one answer per question.

		You've been assigned a project to complete in two weeks. You
	a	get it done right away, even if you have to stay up late.
1	b	procrastinate but finish well at the last minute.
	c	have a challenge finishing as you want the project perfect.
	d	take your time, finishing at an easy pace.
		Friends would describe you as
	a	bold and to the point.
2	b	fun and entertaining.
	c	witty and detail-oriented.
	d	likable and easy going.

You find yourself in a conversation with neighbors or coworkers. You

3	a	laugh sometimes and enjoy joining in.
	b	listen and contribute only when needed.
	c	might interrupt with a solution for most problems.
	d	listen and offer encouragement.

The most important thing to have in life is

4	a	peace.
	b	perfection.
	c	fun.
	d	control.

When it comes to friends, you

5	a	make friends easily.
	b	have little need for friends.
	c	make friends cautiously.
	d	get along with everyone.

When choosing a place to eat, you

6	a	act spontaneously.
	b	change your mind often.
	c	have particular places in mind.
	d	don't have a preference.

Your ideal weekend would include

7	a	traveling to a new place.
	b	having quality time with your spouse or a friend.
	c	learning a new skill.
	d	having a pajama day.

When you are stressed, you

8	a	find a quiet place to rest.
	b	call a friend and go shopping.
	c	get away to a spot where you're alone and can recharge.
	d	exercise more.

If you look in your closet you will see

9	a	all the hangers turned the same way and clothes neatly hung.
	b	bright colors and fun patterns.
	c	trendy outfits with all pieces hanging together.
	d	a lot of comfortable clothes.

When your child is hurting, you

10

a	cry with him or her.
b	wrap your arms around him or her in a big hug.
c	tell him or her to be strong and get back into life.
d	try to make him or her feel better by planning something fun.

When you are in a crowd, you

11

a	enjoy all your new best friends.
b	wish you could hurry up and get home and put your feet up.
c	retreat to the perimeter to talk to someone you already know.
d	work the crowd to identify contacts.

People often say you are

12

a	controlling.
b	fun-loving.
c	encouraging.
d	laid back.

Driving to work, you see a man knock a lady over and flee. You would most likely

13

a	call the police and jump to the lady's aid.
b	park the car, call police, and wait.
c	pass on by hoping she's okay.
d	ask if she is alright and text friends to tell what you saw.

Getting on an elevator to go four floors, you

14

a	waste no time in starting a conversation with those already on.
b	move to the back corner and hope the elevator is fast.
c	smile and stand quietly.
d	push the button for your floor and ask the others which floor they're on.

When unexpected company knocks at your door, you

15

a	turn around and shout "Party!"
b	invite them in and immediately begin tidying up.
c	tell them it's good to see them, but you have a headache.
d	invite them in, control the short visit, then stand and bid them good-bye.

While lying in the hammock by the lake, you

16

a	take a nap easily.
b	make a check-list for errands.
c	invite a friend to join you.
d	have a hard time just lying there.

Your parents are coming for a visit. You

17

a	rush around making sure everything is in place and clean.
b	brief the family on how to act and what to do.
c	decide the house is clean enough.
d	call all the relatives letting them know about the visit.

When given the choice you prefer

18

a	to lead.
b	to serve.
c	to research.
d	to entertain.

When you are sad, you

19

a	read a book.
b	tell a friend.
c	work on a project.
d	take a nap.

When given the opportunity to voice your opinion

20

a	you speak right up.
b	give your opinion and more.
c	choose your words carefully.
d	you say very few words.

If you were a piece of a puzzle, you would be

21

a	the corners.
b	the bright flowers.
c	the straight edges.
d	the background.

In life, you tend to be

22

a	playful.
b	purposeful.
c	powerful.
d	peaceful.

Your car of choice would be

23

a	economical and safe.
b	comfortable and easy to maintain.
c	sporty and fun.
d	stylish and dependable.

You are drawn to

24		
	a	things done the right way.
	b	things done the fast way.
	c	things done the easy way.
	d	things done the fun way.

Which word describes you best at home?

25		
	a	competitive
	b	cautious
	c	committed
	d	carefree

Your co-workers describe you as

26		
	a	results-oriented
	b	service-oriented
	c	detail-oriented
	d	pleasure-oriented

Linking Your Chain

This is your first step in discovering more about who you are. How exciting!

1. Transfer your answers to the scoring key on the following page. Simply look at the letter you marked in the assessment and circle it in the appropriate column.

2. Add the total number circled in each column and enter it at the bottom of the key.

3. Circle the column with the highest number. That is your dominant personality.

4. Many people find that another personality column has a fairly high number. For instance, your score may be 14 in the Mobilizer column, 8 in the Organizer column, and 2 in both the Stabilizer and the Socializer columns. This means you are a strong Mobilizer but also have quite a few Organizer tendencies. It also means that you are not likely to demonstrate many of the Stabilizer or Socializer tendencies.

SCORING KEY

	Mobilizer	Socializer	Stabilizer	Organizer
1	a	b	d	c
2	a	b	d	c
3	c	a	d	b
4	d	c	a	b
5	b	a	d	c
6	c	a	d	b
7	c	a	d	b
8	d	b	a	c
9	c	b	d	a
10	c	d	b	a
11	d	a	b	c
12	a	b	d	c
13	a	d	c	b
14	d	a	c	b
15	d	a	c	b
16	b	c	a	d
17	b	d	c	a
18	a	d	b	c
19	c	b	d	a
20	a	b	d	c
21	a	b	d	c
22	c	a	d	b
23	d	c	b	a
24	b	d	c	a
25	a	d	c	b
26	a	d	b	c
	Mobilizer	Socializer	Stabilizer	Organizer

	Mobilizer	Socializer	Stabilizer	Organizer
Total				

Personality Descriptions

Socializers

Socializers are just that—socializers!

They love a party and seek the fun element in everything they do. Socializers love people and feel very lonely when they are not around them. Quiet time is difficult and often requires great discipline for the socializer personality.

Mobilizers

Mobilizers are the movers and shakers of the world.

They set their goals and then move full speed ahead to accomplish them. Mobilizers make great leaders. You often see them as committee chairs or heads of companies. If you want something done, the mobilizer is a good choice for making that happen.

Organizers

Organizers are rule followers who often get labeled as perfectionists!

Those with this personality may also find it hard to love unconditionally. As a deep thinker, the organizer is often well-grounded in his or her faith. If you need a good listener, the organizer is probably your person!

Stabilizers

Stabilizers are seen as the quiet and relaxed personality.

Other personalities often wish they could live that way! Stabilizers love people yet shy away from conflict and change. This personality enjoys situations where they don't feel pressure or stress.

Wrap up

Want to learn more now that you have discovered your personality? Linked® Quick Guides to Personalities are available through bookstores and online from Bold Vision Books and other sites. Additional Linked® Personality Assessments available from the authors. Linked® Personality Assessment used by permission. All rights reserved. © Linda Gilden and Linda Goldfarb. For questions, speaking engagements, or individual coaching, contact the authors at linda@lindagilden.com (Linda Gilden) and linda@livepowerfullynow.org (Linda Goldfarb).

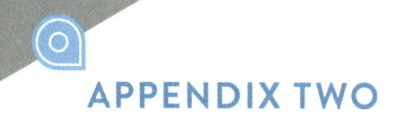

STRENGTHS AND WEAKNESS OF EACH PERSONALITY TYPE

MOBILIZER

STRENGTHS	WEAKNESSES
Born Leader	Bossy
Goal-oriented	Impatient
Strong Willed	Quick-tempered
Decisive	Inflexible
Independent	Domineering
Confident	Knows Everything
Dynamic	May be rude, tactless
Organized	Demands loyalty

STABILIZER

STRENGTHS	WEAKNESSES
Easy Going	Indecisive
Relaxed	Would rather watch
Calm	Too compromising
Competent	Stays uninvolved
Good under pressure	Indifferent
Patient	Judges
Good listener	Resists change
Dry sense of humor	Fearful
Quiet but witty	Worried

SOCIALIZER

STRENGTHS

Storyteller
Sense of humor
Enthusiastic
Cheerful
Makes friends easily
Loves People
Spontaneous
Creative and colorful

WEAKNESSES

Exaggerates
Undisciplined
Easily Distracted
Egotistical
Loud
Wants Center Stage
Wastes time talking
Doesn't listen

ORGANIZER

STRENGTHS

Deep, thoughtful
Analytical
Serious
Perfectionistic
High Standards
Creative
Appreciative of Beauty
Orderly
Economical
Faithful

WEAKNESSES

Moody
Depressed
Low self-image
Deep need for approval
Standards too high
Hard to please
Too Introspective
Guilt feelings
Insecure socially
Withdrawn
Critical of others
Holds back affection

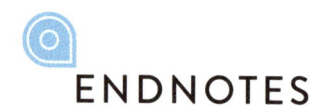

ENDNOTES

[1] Mark Batterson, *Draw the Circle: The 40-Day Prayer Challenge*, Zondervan, 2012.

[2] Ibid.

[3] Jon Bloom, "Lay Aside the Weight of Self-Preoccupation," http://www.desiringgod.org/articles/lay-aside-the-weight-of-self-preoccupation, accessed May 2016.

[4] Geraldine Downey, Ph.D. as quoted by Amanda L. Chan in Huffpost Healthy Living, March 13, 2013.

[5] http://growinghumankindness.com/need-that-drives-overeating/, accessed November 2015.

[6] Concept of percentage forgiving adapted from *When He Leaves* by Kari West and Noelle Quinn (Eugene, OR: Harvest House Publishers, 1998).

[7] http://rickwarren.org/devotional/english/you-were-made-for-relationship, accessed October 2015.

[8] Claire Messud, *The Woman Upstairs* (New York: Random House LLC, 2013).

[9] Georgia Shaffer, www.georgiashaffer.com.

[10] http://www.medicaldaily.com/you-are-what-you-eat-how-personality-traits-can-influence-weight-326342, accessed May 2016.

[11] Anonymous.

[12] http://www.barefootsworld.net/aaresentments.html, accessed October 2015.

[13] Alice May, *Surviving Betrayal* (New York: HarperSanFrancisco, 1999).